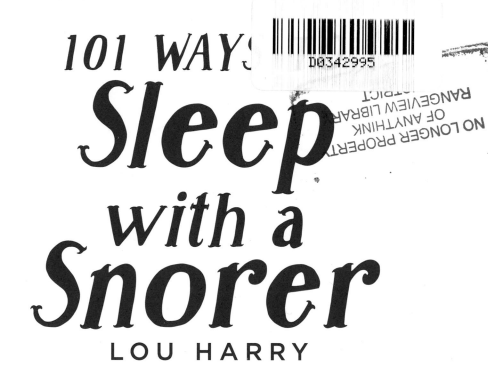

101 WAYS *Sleep* with a *Snorer*

LOU HARRY

Cider Mill Press
Kennebunkport, Maine

NO LONGER PROPERTY OF ANYTHINK RANGEVIEW LIBRARY DISTRICT

101 Ways to Sleep with a Snorer
Copyright © 2017 by Appleseed Press Book
Publishers LLC.

This is an officially licensed book by Cider Mill
Press Book Publishers LLC.

All rights reserved under the Pan-American and
International Copyright Conventions.

No part of this book may be reproduced in whole
or in part, scanned, photocopied, recorded,
distributed in any printed or electronic form, or
reproduced in any manner whatsoever, or by any
information storage and retrieval system now
known or hereafter invented, without express
written permission of the publisher, except in
the case of brief quotations embodied in critical
articles and reviews.

The scanning, uploading, and distribution of
this book via the Internet or via any other means
without permission of the publisher is illegal and
punishable by law. Please support authors' rights,
and do not participate in or encourage piracy of
copyrighted materials.

13-Digit ISBN: 978-1604337211
10-Digit ISBN: 1604337214

This book may be ordered by mail from the
publisher. Please include $5.99 for postage and
handling. Please support your local bookseller
first!

Books published by Cider Mill Press Book
Publishers are available at special discounts
for bulk purchases in the United States
by corporations, institutions, and other
organizations. For more information, please
contact the publisher.

Cider Mill Press Book Publishers
"Where good books are ready for press"
PO Box 454
12 Spring Street
Kennebunkport, Maine 04046

Visit us on the Web!
www.cidermillpress.com

Cover and interior design by Debbie Berne
Illustrations by Alex Kalomeris
All other images and vectors used under official
license from Shutterstock.com

Printed in China
1 2 3 4 5 6 7 8 9 0
First Edition

for Cindy
Who suffered long enough before
I strapped on the CPAP.

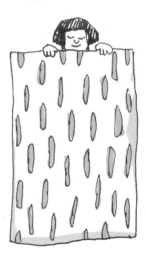

Contents

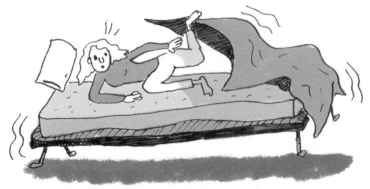

Introduction

IT'S BEEN A long day. You've done your best to meet the world's expectations of you. You've tried to make it a better place—or, at least, not a worse one. You've worked hard to balance the interests of yourself, your family, your friends, and others you encounter throughout the day.

Now it's time for sleep.

And you're lying next to a foghorn.

Granted, you love this foghorn. But you also know you need your sleep. Forget beauty rest—you need getting-through-the-day rest. But that earth-shattering sound coming from the other side of the bed is going to make that impossible. There are enough challenges for any relationship during traditional waking hours to have to deal with more during traditional sleeping hours.

What to do?

Well, while I can't vouch for every effort made to keep snoring at bay, I have collected 101 different ways to address the problem, from the silly to the surgical. Some are questionable home remedies passed down through generations; others are over-the-counter efforts to lower the volume in your bedroom.

Good luck.

And good night.

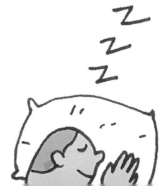

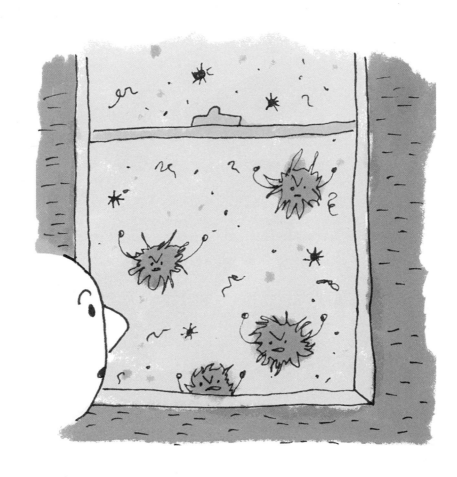

№ 1

Close the Window

GETTING RID OF airborne irritants (and I don't mean that person monopolizing the armrest next to you on the plane) can be an easy solution to simple snoring. Closing the window—combined with dusting—can go a long way toward reducing the causes. If nothing else, it might make it easier for the neighbors to sleep.

№ 2

Pile Pillows

THE HIGHER THE head, the less likely contact will be made between throat tissues. Thank gravity for that. And an extra pillow—or three, or four—can be enough to open one's breathing airway and keep the tongue from blocking the throat. Be warned, though: Propping someone up too high can actually cause snoring. If you need immediate relief in the middle of the night, place a hand under the snorer's neck and gently tilt their head to avoid waking them.

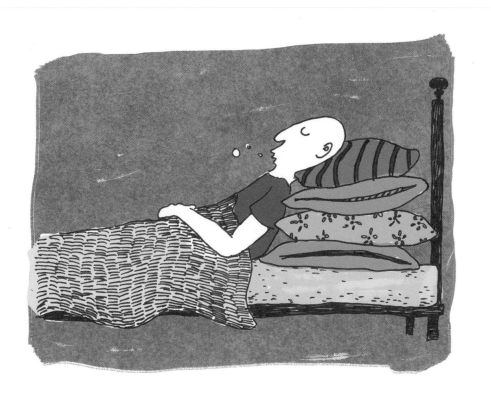

№ 3

Raise the Head of the Bed

A FIRMER, MORE consistent version of the pillow pile, raising the head of your bed is only an option with certain types of beds—unless you want to tilt the entire thing, which puts you at risk of sliding off, which would be difficult to explain to the EMTs. If both bedmates don't want the tilt, split beds are also an option. Bonus: In this position, it's easier to watch TV. Downside: It's tempting to watch *more* TV.

Nº 4

Change the Pillows

LET'S BE CLEAR, this does not mean tossing your partner's pillow in the guest room and taking out replacements from the closet. It means ditching the pillows completely and replacing them with new ones. Still resistant? Think about the fact that the old pillows may be home to millions of dust mites, which have been known to contribute to allergies. That image might ease the transition for you.

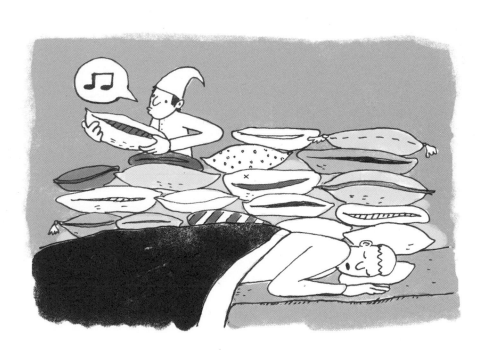

№ 5

Build a Pillow Barricade

IT DOESN'T HAVE pillow-piling's physiological value, sure, but a pillow barricade between you and the offending sleeper can provide some sound reduction and help you get to sleep. Okay, so it's about as effective as the barricade created by the student resistance fighters in *Les Misérables*, and that didn't end well. But there is a positive: If you are tempted to lash out at the snorer, the pillow barricade provides a level of physical protection.

Nº 6

Use a Body Pillow

BODY PILLOWS—PILLOWS the length of the body, designed to aid fibromyalgia patients but also popular with pregnant women—have a history of assisting chronic back pain (and occasional loneliness). But these oversized creations can take up as much room on the bed as you do. The advantage is that they can also help your partner stay on their side while sleeping, which helps mitigate mild snoring in a way that's much more stable than a pillow mountain. Downside: You'll need a complete, separate set of pillowcases.

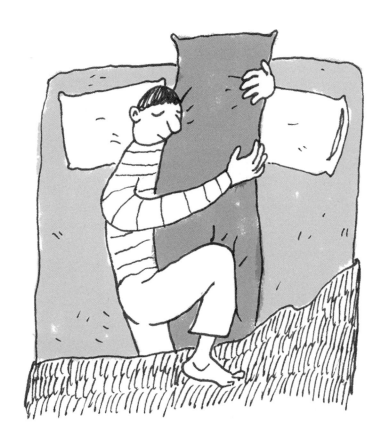

Nº 7

Use a Firmer Pillow

BEFORE YOU BUY just any pillow, though, maximize your chances of success with one that doesn't offer much resistance. Of course, your partner may resist the very idea of it—some people like sinking so deep into their pillow that it practically covers their ears. But the firmer the pillow the stronger the support, and the better the chance of reduced snoring.

№ 8

Switch to Anti-Snore Pillows

THERE ARE MANY pillows out there specifically marketed for their alleged ability to fight snoring. And while some anecdotal evidence supports those claims, these products have plenty of disappointed user reviews too. These memory-foam pillows may still help back- and side-sleepers, provided the sleeper nods off in such a way that their chin is lifted away from the chest. Just be careful of the ones that promise to eliminate snoring completely.

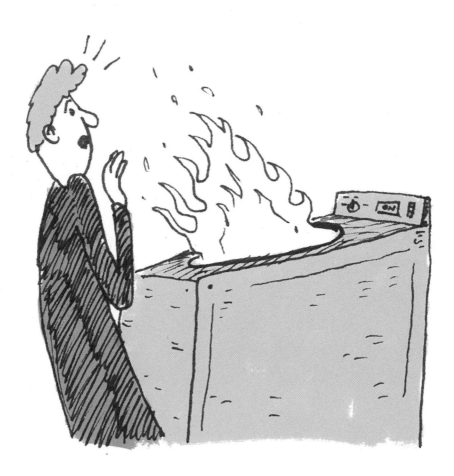

№ 9

Wash Pillowcases in Hot Water

ON WASH DAY, it may be easier to just throw the pillowcases in with everything else and turn the dial to cold as usual. Yes, that will effectively separate your colors. But unfortunately it won't do much to kill the dust mites hanging out on the pillowcases. Kick it up to hot for a better clean . . . and possibly a better night's sleep.

Nº 10

Get Zippered Pillowcases

TO BUILD ON the previous pillow ideas, look into purchasing zippered pillowcases when upgrading your head support. The zipper's extra protection helps keep out those dust mites and extend the pillow's life. Bonus: You can hide extra cash there without worrying it will fall out. (Okay, there goes that secret.)

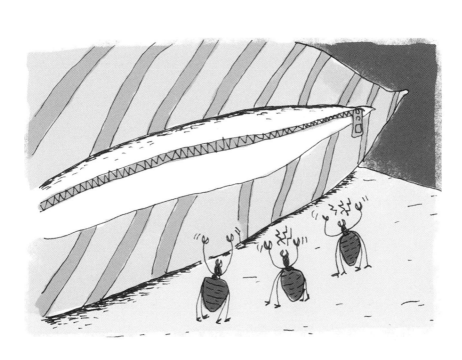

№ 11

Relocate to the Spare Bedroom or Living Room Couch

HAVING A GETAWAY room in your domicile is a plus for multiple reasons— and indicates a certain degree of financial achievement (congrats). Of course, you can't live in exile for the rest of your relationship. Remember that this is just a temporary solution; it may result in a good night's sleep, but it also risks permanent self-exile once you remember the pleasures of sleeping alone. And yes, the living room couch may be a comfortable spot to watch television. That's why you bought it, right? But relocating to the bedroom equivalent of the suburbs is just another temporary solution for those who don't have a spare bedroom. Downside: You could find yourself awake as ever, only binge-watching a TV series instead of listening to incessant snoring. Upside: You'll have more to talk about during the day . . . assuming you can stay awake at work. And hey, separate beds worked on black and white TV shows—just look at an episode of *The Dick Van Dyke Show* (recommended regardless of your reason). If separate beds are good enough for Rob and Laura Petrie, they might be tolerable for you and your partner.

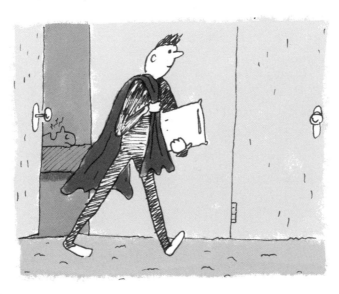

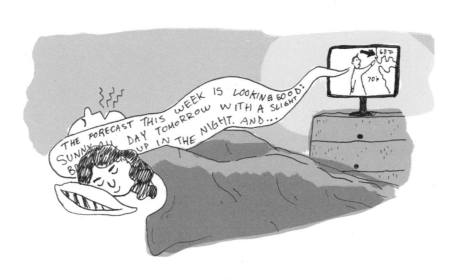

№ 12

Turn On the TV

PUMPING UP THE volume can serve two purposes. First, it will drown out some of your bedmate's incessant noise. Second, it may wake said bedmate up. The downside is that it can keep you awake as well, leading to an even groggier morning.

№ 13

Clean Your Room

DON'T TAKE THIS as a judgment of any kind, but there's a chance that your bedroom isn't as clean as it could be. You don't need an investigative team with infrared cameras to know that dust, pet dander, pollen, and more are probably floating around your abode. And these congestion-causers may be contributing to the snoring. It won't help you tonight, but vacuuming tomorrow could lead to more restful nights.

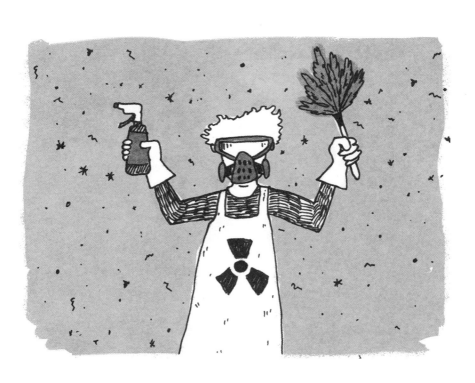

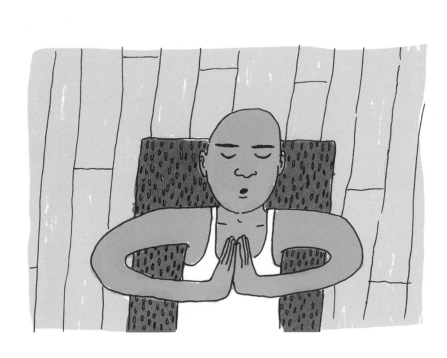

№ 14

Try Yoga

THERE ARE A number of exercises that yoga enthusiasts claim will open your airways and reduce sleep-honking. Popular among them is *Pranayama*, a breathing exercise that hardly feels like exercise at all. The snorer simply sits on the mat with a straight back, breathes in deeply, holds for three seconds and exhales. *Brahmari*, a variation, involves breathing from the stomach and, when exhaling, making a humming, bee-like sound. A bit more involved is *Ujjayi Pranayama*, in which you breathe deeply through one nostril then exhale assertively through the other. Of course, these should be done *before* going to bed.

№ 15

Adorn Yourself with Earplugs

THE SIMPLEST OF low-tech wonders can block out the noise, but keep in mind that they'll also block out your alarm clock. Missing once might not be a problem—and a good night's sleep may actually lead to more productivity in the long run. But as snoring is an ongoing problem, so too will be your chronic lateness to work. Or consider earmuffs. There are a wide variety of earmuffs on the market, but they have one thing in common: They aren't designed to keep out sound, just to keep out the cold. While some models are denser than others, the reality is that these aren't very effective in the bedroom. Unless your partner is into that, which has nothing to do with snoring.

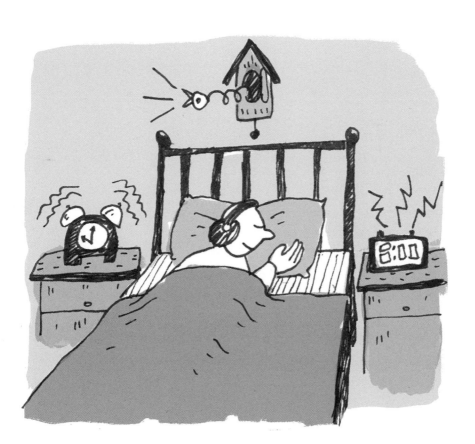

№ 16

Try a Headset

SIMILAR TO THE aforementioned earplugs, a headset gives you the option of listening to something you prefer to the log-sawing. The same missing-the-alarm danger that applies to earplugs also applies here, although newer headset models solve that problem with built-in alarm capability. Ain't technology grand?

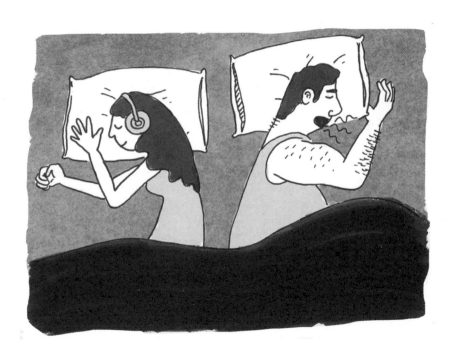

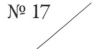

Nº 17

Do the Side-Shift

SNORING IS OFTEN accentuated when the sleeper lies face-up. Shifting the snorer from their back to their side can help, at least temporarily. One option is the arm-pull, in which you grab the snorer's far-side arm and pull it toward you. The downside here is that if it doesn't work—if the side position is obtained but the problem continues—the snorer is now snoring in your direction. More difficult is the standard push, which requires lots of force combined with upward pressure so that you don't just shove the snorer off the bed.

Nº 18

Apply a Neck Brace

GOT A NECK brace lying around from the last time you had whiplash? Slap it around your partner's neck and it could keep the chin extended enough to keep the airway open. Just remember to remove it in the morning—unless getting sympathy at work is also part of the plan.

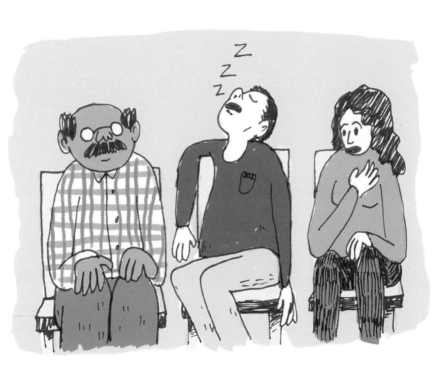

№ 19

Join a Support Group

YES, THERE ARE Facebook groups, meet-ups, and doctor-sponsored get-to-gethers for partners of snorers. If nothing else, you'll know that you aren't alone. And if the other attendees have boring stories, you might be able to catch some zzz's at the gathering.

№ 20

Take a Shower

HITTING THE SHOWERS before hitting the hay not only keeps the sheets cleaner—and encourages more playful activity because, you know, you smell better—it also helps open those nasal passages. Of course, depending on how much of that playful activity you engage in, a second shower may be in order, which cuts down on your sleep time.

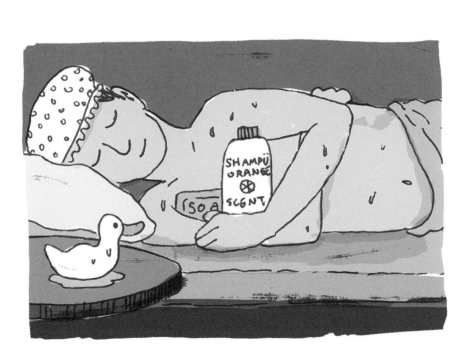

№ 21

Cut Out Pre-Sleep Snacks and Late-Evening Meals

THINKING ABOUT SOME late-night dining? Think again. The very act of digestion relaxes the tongue and throat muscles, which contributes to snoring, so best to get eating out of the way when the rest of the world has dinner and not just before bed. This will also help with weight loss, another possible snoring cure.

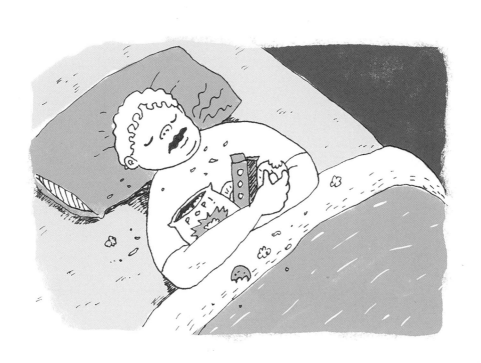

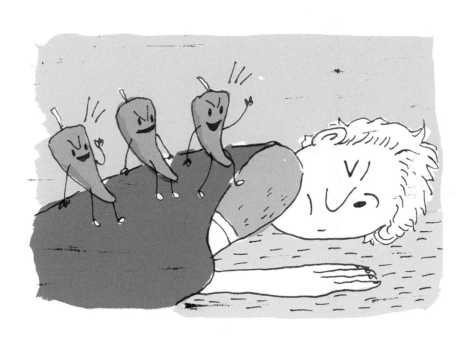

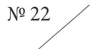

Nº 22

Avoid Spicy and Fatty Foods

IN ADDITION TO eating wisely before bedtime, snorers should be careful about what they consume any time of day. Spicy foods can lead to indigestion, which can in turn lead to snoring. Ditto for fatty foods that cause heartburn. Craving those foods? Try shifting them into your lunchtime rotation.

Nº 23

Upgrade the Exercise Regimen

NOW COMES THE tough love. There have been countless studies that prove higher weight increases one's chance of snoring. Getting on an effective weight-loss regimen reduces—and sometimes cures—snoring. This long-term solution may not help you get sleep tonight, but it will lead to a much more restful life.

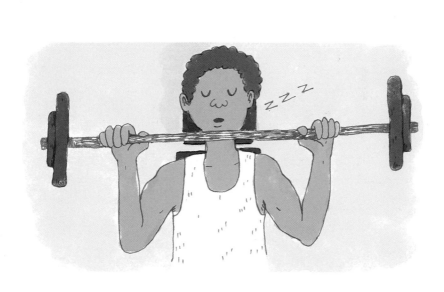

№ 24

Lose Neck Weight

IF YOUR PARTNER isn't quite ready or disciplined enough to lose weight, a more focused approach—specifically to neck fat—could help. Snorenation.com offers some excellent tips, but a simple web search will find a host of other exercises, many of which can be performed while working at a desk or sitting in a waiting room. Just prepare for co-workers to ask, "Are you okay?"

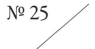

№ 25

Smart Beds

SOME HIGH-END BEDS not only adjust to your comfort but can also track your sleep patterns. While they claim to help snoring, usually these fall into the "temporary relief for minor snoring" category. That said, just being able to adjust snorers six degrees or so might make a difference, provided sleep apnea isn't the core cause.

№ 26

Quit Smoking

NO, NOT YOU—your bed partner. Although it wouldn't be a bad thing for you, either. Smoking irritates the nose and throat, blocking airways and worsening the snoring problem. While the ideal is to have never started smoking in the first place, the best approach is to quit now.

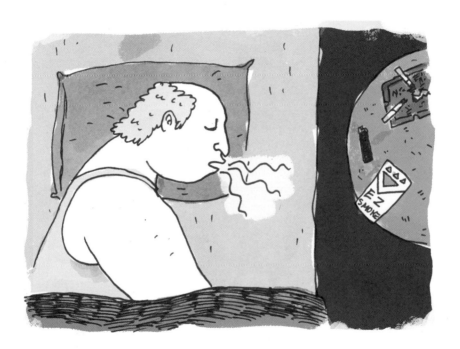

Nº 27

Use a Humidifier

ADDING SOME MOISTURE to the air via an electronic device can make a difference for some snorers, particularly those living in a dry climate. Before you run out and buy a humidifier, though, make sure you are clear on one thing: A dehumidifier is a very different device. Quite the opposite, in fact!

Nº 28

Add Peppermint Oil to the Humidifier

FOR A GENTLER version of the previous tip—and a room that offers a holiday scent—add a few drops of peppermint oil to your humidifier about a half hour before you hit the sack. Its anti-inflammatory properties will help keep that airway open.

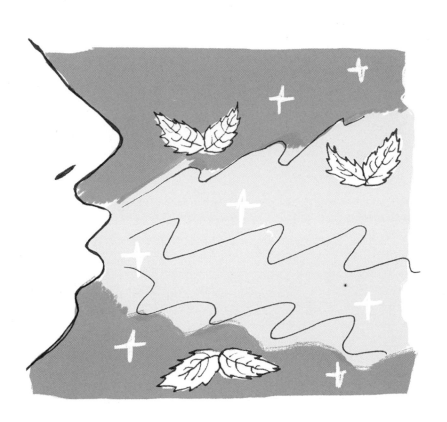

№ 29

Gargle with Peppermint Mouthwash

WHILE BY NO means a long-term solution, a swig, swish, and spit of peppermint mouthwash before bed can help temporarily shrink mouth tissue. Side effect: A minty mouth will also make the goodnight kiss just a little bit sweeter.

№ 30

Train Your Uvula

YES, YOU READ that right. And just to prove this isn't made up, try this exercise: Open your mouth, contract the muscle at the back of your throat, and repeat for 30 seconds. Do it in front of a mirror and you should see the uvula moving. If nothing else, you can say it happened.

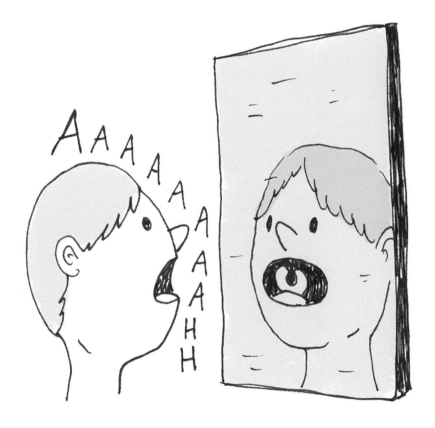

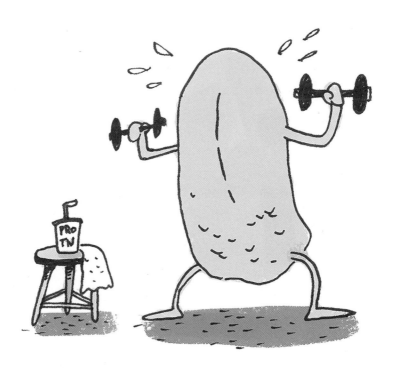

№ 31

Give Your Tongue a Workout

WHY SHOULD YOUR uvula have all the fun? Here's one your open-to-things-that-sound-crazy partner may want to try: Find the top of your front teeth with the tip of your tongue. Slide the tongue backwards and forwards for about three minutes a day.

Nº 32

Exercise Your Jaw

HERE'S ANOTHER THROAT exercise to add to your partner's repertoire: Open the mouth and move the jaw to one side. Keep it there for about half a minute, then do the same on the other side.

Nº 33

Avoid Alcohol

THAT NIGHTCAP CAN help your partner get to sleep—alcohol has been known to do that—but it might also keep you awake by relaxing their airway muscles. Unfortunately, if you're reading this in bed, there's no way to de-alcohol someone tonight. But if you see a correlation between nips and snores going forward, cut out the post-dinner indulgence.

Nº 34

Sing

NO KIDDING. WITH findings based on a U.K. study, there's actually a "Singing for Snorers" program (singingforsnorers.com) offering exercises designed to aid those with mild-to-moderate apnea. But be warned: Even though it was on its fourth edition as of 2017, the program's designers make clear that it's still part of a study and results are not guaranteed. Still, at least there will be more music in your life.

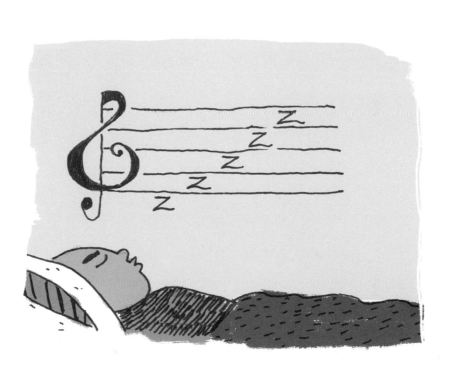

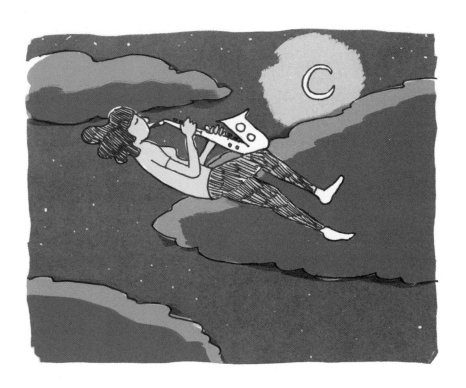

№ 35

Take Up a
Musical Instrument

NO, A GUITAR or piano won't help you. But playing a clarinet, flute, or other wind instrument can positively impact your throat muscles. Bonus possibility: Your partner starts getting gigs that prevent them from coming home until you're already asleep.

№ 36

Stabilize Your Bed

IT MAY NOT be the snoring that wakes you up but rather the movement of your bed *caused* by the snorer. A mini-quake may not show up on the Richter scale, but a shake here and there can be enough to bring you to consciousness. If your bed isn't on firm footing, some adjustment could eliminate that shaking. If you can't get your standard metal frame to comply—or don't trust yourself balancing the short leg on unread books—consider a platform bed frame.

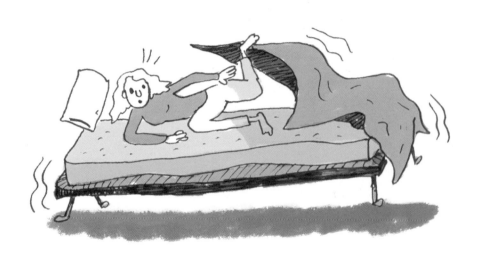

Nº 37

Try Compression Socks

RESEARCHERS HAVE FOUND that wearing compression socks during the day lowers the amount of fluid in one's lower legs. Less fluid in the legs means less fluid is likely to move up the body to the neck, which can cause snoring. Plus your feet will stay toasty.

Nº 38

Get Magnetized

ONE BRAND OF snore reducers, Snoreclipse, makes a device that uses magnets to apply pressure on the septum and free up airways. When inserted, it looks like the wearer is sporting a tiny nose ring. Bonus: Thanks to the magnets, you might attract some loose chain that fell out in your bed.

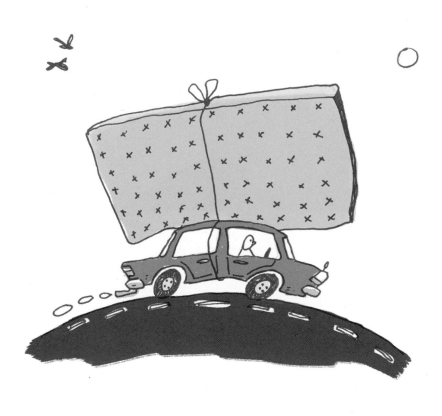

№ 39

Get a Bigger Bed

A BIGGER BED always helps in a snoring crisis. The more floor space your bed covers, the more room you have to move to the far side—and the less likely you are to feel every vibration your partner causes.

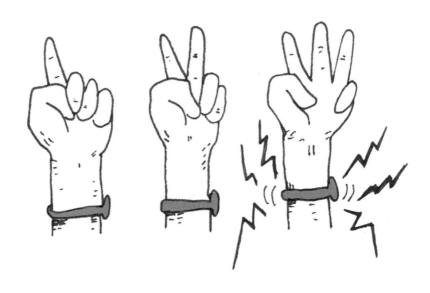

№ 40

Snore Stopper

DON'T BE SHOCKED. Well, actually, your partner will be a little shocked by this device, which straps onto the wrist and emits an electric jolt after detecting three loud noises in a row. The intensity can be adjusted to the snorer's preference; the idea isn't to wake them, just to temporarily tense their throat muscles.

№ 41

Upgrade Your Mattress

JUST AS REPLACING your old pillows can decrease snoring, so can replacing a mattress (albeit at a significantly higher price). And if it doesn't, well, you've wanted a better mattress anyway. But you may not need to take the drastic—and costly—step of ditching your whole mattress; you can also try upgrading your mattress cover (or getting one in the first place, if you don't already have one). The new cover should help absorb vibrations caused by the human wind tunnel next to you.

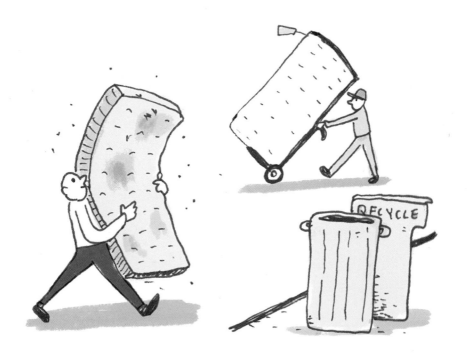

№ 42

Create a Sleep Pattern

ERRATIC SLEEP PATTERNS—early to bed one night, late to bed another—can contribute to snoring. While it's not always possible to make life perfectly consistent (and who would want that?), it's still useful to zero in on a bed time and try to stick to it whenever possible.

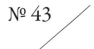

Nº 43

Recite Your Vowels

SOME RECOMMEND RECITING the vowels—a, e, i, o, u (you can skip the y)—for several minutes several times a day to strengthen the muscles in the upper respiratory tract. Stay consonant—er, consistent—and snoring may be reduced.

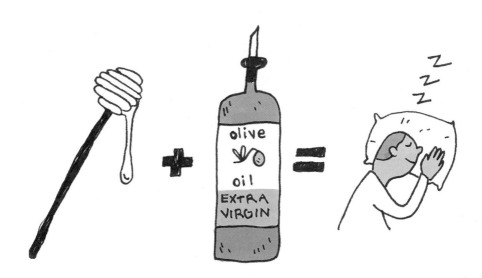

Nº 44

Try Some Olive Oil

YOU CAN REDUCE mild snoring by taking a few sips of olive oil before bed—either straight or mixed with honey. Why? The general theory posits that olive oil lubricates tissues in the back of the throat, reducing the chance of vibration. Additionally, olive oil's anti-inflammatory properties can reduce swelling and tighten the muscles under the palate.

Nº 45

Offer a Bit of Clarified Butter

THERE ARE SOME home remedy advocates who swear by clarified butter, or ghee, made from cow's milk. With roots traced back to ancient India, ghee is still used to treat a variety of ailments in South Asian and Arabic countries. Warm some up, apply a drop into each of the snorer's nostrils before bedtime and, in the morning, see if you're a convert.

Nº 46

Incorporate the Cardamom

SOME CALL IT cardamom. Some call it cardamon. Hopefully you'll call it a lifesaver (or at least a nightsaver). Advocates recommend adding a teaspoon in powdered form to warm water and drinking a half hour before bed to open blocked nasal passages.

Nº 47

Tap the Turmeric

ANOTHER HERBAL EFFORT involves this main spice in curry, a lesser-known relative of ginger found primarily in southern Asia. Adding two teaspoons of turmeric powder to a glass of milk before bed can reduce inflammation in the throat and airways, per top10homeremedies.com.

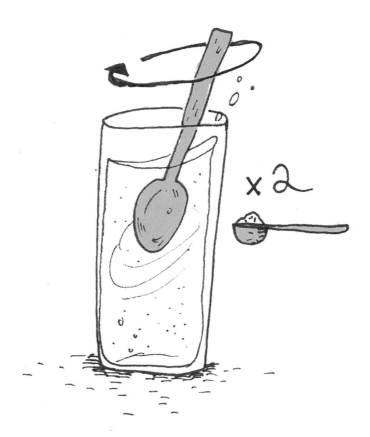

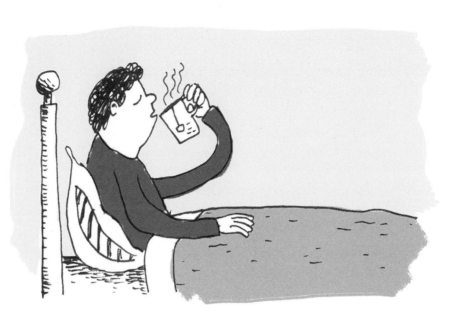

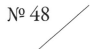

Nº 48

Nettle Leaf Tea

WHILE IT'S UNLIKELY to topple Earl Grey in the pantheon of top teas, nettle leaf tea is recommended by homeremedyhacks.com and other herbal remedy sites to treat snoring. Primarily for those with seasonal allergies, the recommended dosage is three cups daily to reduce the inflammation caused by pollen and other allergens. Any less, and you won't know for sure if the remedy is working.

№ 49

Avoid Milk

NOBODY SAID SNORERS were consistent. While the aforementioned turmeric approach required milk, sometimes consuming milk or dairy products can contribute to the problem by increasing mucus production—and thicker-than-normal mucus to boot. Try cutting it out in the evening and consume your calcium in the morning instead.

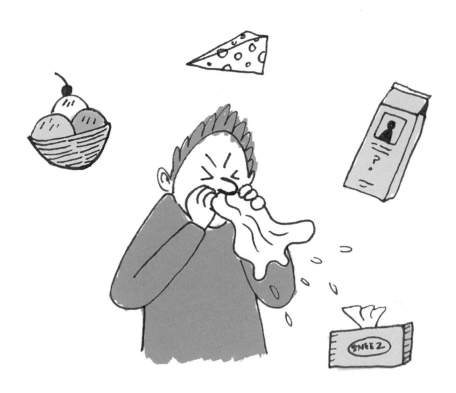

№ 50

CPAP Machine

THE INITIALS STAND for continuous positive airway pressure, and while lugging around the equipment on business trips and vacations can be a pain (although medical equipment doesn't count toward your airline carry-on limit), the device is effective on apnea patients. It keeps pressurized air flowing through the snorer's airways thanks to a tightly-sealed mask and some even allow techs to monitor your sleep patterns, transmitting reports directly from the machine.

№ 51

Extend the Cord

FOR SOME, THE CPAP machine is a lifesaver—but the noise of the machine itself can end up keeping you awake. The solution? Some CPAP manufacturers offer extended tubes that allow you to keep the machine further away.

Nº 52

Hydrate

YES, THERE ARE plenty of home remedy herbal drinks that you can try. But the H_2Obvious answer is to just drink your water straight. Dehydration can create sticky, thick mucus in the nose, which contributes to snoring. Or hydrate with less water. For some reason, some people are resistant to the idea of guzzling water. These folks should explore other options, such as water-based soups, gelatin, and sports drinks (in moderation).

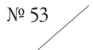

№ 53

Seal the Deal

CLOSING THE MOUTH is actually the thinking behind devices like the Snore Seal, a disposable anti-snoring creation that cuts down on air intake through the mouth but still allows exhaling. It kind of looks like the snorer is trying to play the world's smallest harmonica.

№ 54

Cut the Caffeine

WHETHER IN COFFEE, soda, a chocolate bar, or those little bottles that give you the boost you crave, caffeine is America's favorite stimulant. But caffeine can cause your body to lose water. And dehydration—we've been through this—causes snoring. Another problem: Snorers sleeping poorly may gravitate toward more caffeine to make up for the lack of sleep, creating a vicious cycle.

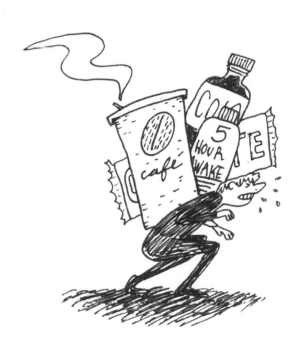

No 55

Dip Into a Neti Pot

THE NETI POT is a nasal irrigation system that rinses the sinuses with warm salt water. Water, salt, and baking soda are mixed in the pot and then the spout is placed in each nostril, draining through the other. Be sure to use sterilized or distilled water when you try it. And don't overload the salt!

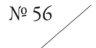

№ 56

Attach a Breathe Right Strip

EVEN THOUGH THEY feel like a Band-Aid over one's nose, Breathe Right nasal strips became a phenomenon in part because of their popularity among football players during games. Rather than using chemistry, the strips rely on physiology, attempting to reduce or eliminate snoring by gently pulling the air passages open.

№ 57

Try a Theravent or Another Nasal Strip

A BREATHE RIGHT variant, Theravent uses what the company calls "MicroValves" to help open and close the airway. They've also got a Theravent Light version—for light snorers, not the calorie-conscious. Of course, given the simplicity of the Breathe Right design, there are plenty of similarly, named variations that do the same thing. You'll know pretty quickly if you've found a cheaper-but-equal one or one with minimal staying (on your nose) power.

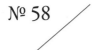

Nº 58

Go with Provent

PROVENT CLAIMS TO help sleep apnea snorers by increasing the exhale pressure, using the snorer's own breathing. Still looking for a major difference? Well, these cover the nostrils themselves. Each has a small hole, so that snorers have no trouble breathing in but face some resistance breathing out, forcing a wider airway. Just be careful about sneezing.

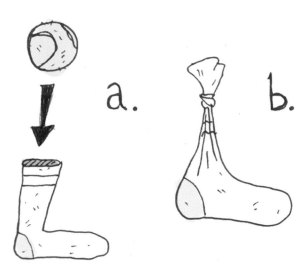

a.

b.

Nº 59

Attempt the Old Sock-and-Tennis-Ball Trick

HERE'S THE IDEA: Drop a tennis ball in a sock and attach it to the back of whatever torso-covering garment the snorer wears to sleep. This should keep them from back-sleeping and keep them on their side—a position less likely to induce honking. Of course, you'll need to fight the temptation to whack your partner with the sock if it doesn't work.

Nº 60

Update Your Air Filter

IT'S EASY TO forget how often you are supposed to change the filter on your home heating and air conditioning unit. (Short answer: Way more often than you probably do.) Switching out the air filter will clean the air more effectively and hopefully reduce the throat irritation that leads to snoring. It can also extend the life of your heater or air conditioner.

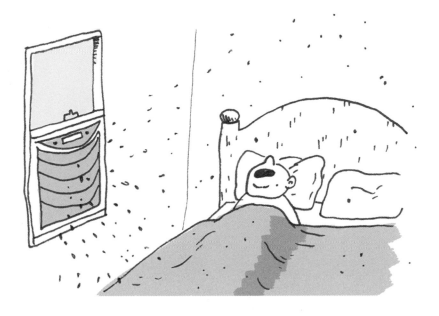

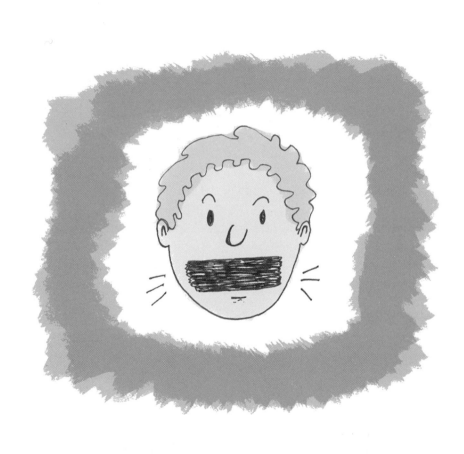

№ 61

Tape Their Mouth

IT SOUNDS HARSH, but some couples have resorted to taping the snorer's mouth. The idea is to force the snorer to breathe through their nose.

№ 62

Tickle

YOU MAY BE tempted to shove, elbow, or push when confronted with a snorer. But how about tickling instead? No, not a "make 'em laugh" tickle—just a gentle tickling of the hair on the neck. Believing it's an itch, the snorer may wake up for a bit to scratch, change sleep positions and, hopefully, give you enough time to fall sleep before the snoring starts again.

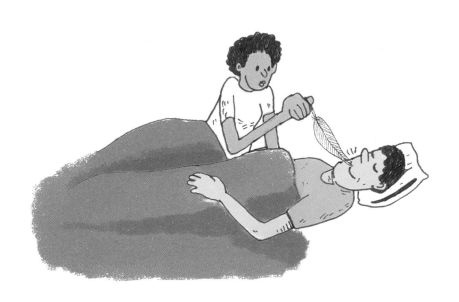

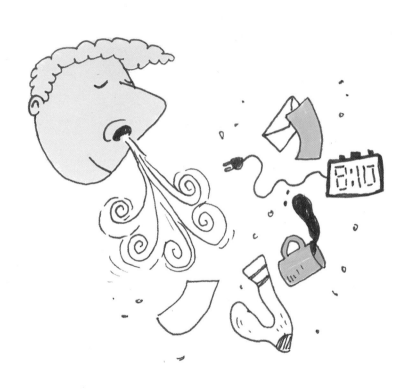

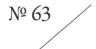

Nº 63

Apply a Nose Clip

THESE DEVICES ARE essentially the plastic inverse of a clothespin over the nose. With two ends inserted into the nostrils, nose clips address minor snoring issues by holding each channel open, making breathing easier . . . and quieter. If you try one of these, such as the Snorepin, take the recommended daily cleaning *very* seriously.

№ 64

Airmax

LIKE THE NOSE clip, the latex-free Airmax is inserted into the nose. Once in, it pushes against the outer part of each nostril, widening it in order to expand the narrowest parts of the nasal passages. The manufacturer claims that Airmax can be used with a CPAP for double protection.

№ 65

Submit to Allergy Tests

BELIEVE IT OR not, medical science actually has a handle on some of the issues that lead to snoring. Haven't been tested lately? Or ever? The snorer in your life could be the victim of very nasty allergies. Wouldn't it be wonderful if relief were just a few shots away?

№ 66

White Noise Machine

DESIGNED TO EVEN out the sound in a room, a white noise machine probably won't drown your partner out completely. But these sound conditioners generate a continuous tone that can make sleeping easier. If you'd like something a bit more atmospheric, some devices provide you with ocean waves or bird chirps rather than the generic white noise.

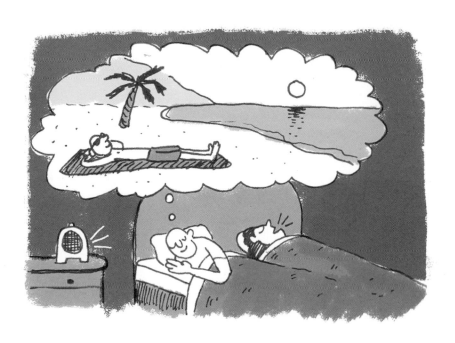

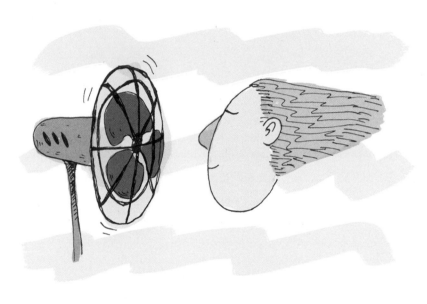

Turn On the Fan or Turn Up the AC

A SIMPLE ROTATING fan can serve a purpose similar to that of the white noise machine—although it offers fewer sound variations. While slightly more expensive to run than fans, air conditioners are also good substitutes for white noise machines. Even better, they help filter out airborne irritants. Just make sure you don't compensate for the cold by dragging an old blanket out of the closet—it may be packed with its own irritants.

№ 68

Try Separate Blankets

IF YOU SHARE a blanket that covers the entire bed, you are at the mercy of the twists and turns of your partner. But with separate blankets, you can roll yourself up in yours and have an easier time pulling it over your head to buffer the sound. Separate blankets may add a step to making the bed in the morning, but they could help you get through the night.

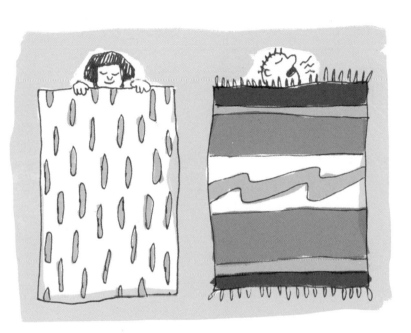

Sport a Mandibular Advancement Device

THESE ORAL APPLIANCES (a phrase that will never, ever sound okay) move the mandible forward, holding the collapsible part of the airway open. They can also help strengthen the airway walls. Just take care of the good night kiss first.

№ 70

Try Palatal Implants

ALSO KNOWN AS the Pillar Procedure (which sounds like a John Ludlum novel), this process involves building up the soft palate by reinforcing it with plastic implants. The goal is to cut down on tissue vibration, and it only takes about 20 minutes under a local anesthetic.

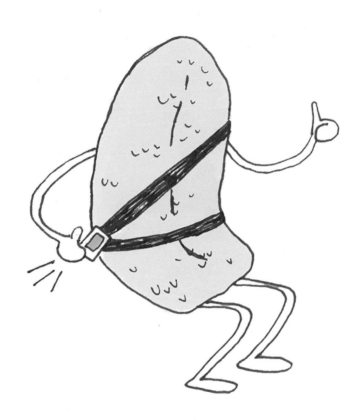

№ 71

Hold Your Tongue

IF IT'S SITTING on your desk, the Zyppah—a variation of the aforementioned mandibular advancement device—might be mistaken for a staple remover. It's actually a mouth guard gadget that, according to the marketing materials, is "like a seatbelt for your tongue," moving the jaw forward and stabilizing the tongue so it doesn't block the airway. When these folks say, "Hold your tongue," they really mean it.

№ 72

Take an Oral Decongestant

THE POINT OF a decongestant is to narrow the blood vessels, minimizing blood supply to the mucus membranes. If nasal decongestion is the cause of the snoring, an over-the-counter (or behind-the-counter, depending on where you live) nasal or pill decongestant such as Afrin or Sudafed could do the trick. Just don't think of this as a permanent solution as nasal decongestants shouldn't be used more than three days in a row.

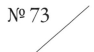

№ 73

Palate Strips

UNLIKE BREATHE RIGHT and other nasal strips, these strips—marketed under names such as Snorisol—don't go on the nose but inside the mouth. Attached to the hard palate, they moisten the hard and soft palate as they dissolve and, per the manufacturers, tighten the tissue and minimize vibrations. However, they aren't meant to be used by those with sleep apnea.

№ 74

Install Blackout Curtains

WHEN YOU ARE kept awake by snoring, everything else in the room can be an eye-opening distraction. Room-darkening curtains can help—though there's also the chance that cutting out all visual input makes you focus more on the snoring, worsening matters.

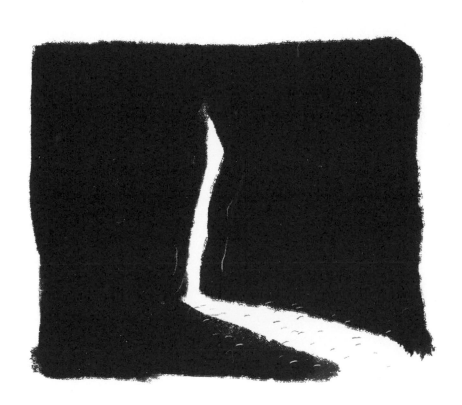

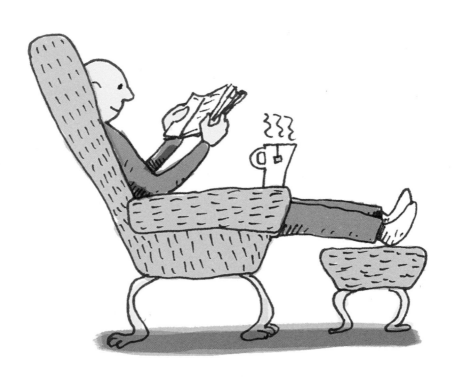

Nº 75

Meditate and Relax

SNORING IS ANNOYING, no question about it. But for some, the anger and resentment snoring causes can do as much damage as the sound itself. Does this "Power of Positive Thinking" approach actually work? If your attitude toward fellow humans leans toward "Gandhi-esque," this budget-conscious approach is worth trying.

Nº 76

Strap On a Chin Strap

IF YOU DON'T mind your snorer looking like they're ready for a college wrestling match, this is a possible solution. Marketed under such names as SnoreX, SnoreShield, and SnoreDoc, these hold the jaw in a forward position, reducing the chance of tongue and throat tissue covering the airway.

№ 77

Stop Grinding Teeth

WHILE THIS MAY seem like a different noisy annoyance, grinding one's teeth at night can contribute to snoring by pushing the tongue back toward the throat. Mouth guards are the obvious solution here, but drinking more water, cutting out gum, and trying to relax one's face during the day can help as well.

Nº 78

Zap the Turbinates

SWOLLEN SINUS TURBINATES can cause nasal blockage, which can in turn cause snoring. When home remedies and medication don't do the job, this in-office procedure might. It's generally used to address severe allergies, but reduced snoring can be a positive side effect. It's a quickie procedure under local anesthetic using a radio frequency–emitting wand—a thin probe inserted into the nose to shrink the turbinate tissue.

№ 79

Take Out the Tissue

USED TO REMOVE throat tissue, UPPP surgery—or uvulopalato-pharyngoplasty—widens the airway. This can include the uvula, tonsils, and adenoids, as well as tissue from the roof of the mouth. Afterward, you can look forward to about three weeks of recovery time and a very sore throat (bring on the ice cream). Remember, though, that surgery is a pretty drastic step and is rarely used solely to eliminate snoring.

№ 80

Somnoplasty

WHILE WE'RE ON the subject of surgical procedures, here's one that's usually performed under local anesthesia. In it, low doses of radio frequency heat are used to remove tissue from the soft palate and uvula.

№ 81

Balloon Sinuplasty

YET ANOTHER SURGICAL procedure, this addresses sinus-related snoring and is usually performed by an ear, nose, and throat specialist using a wire and flexible balloon. When the balloon is inflated, it opens up the sinuses. Saline is sprayed in to clear out pus and mucus, and the balloon is removed. A plus: No cutting involved.

Nº 82

Remove the Uvula

WHEN THE UVULA flaps around, snoring can occur (so can a sore throat). Remove the uvula and the snoring problem might go away. But don't try doing this at home. It's called a uvulectomy (of course) and you can figure out for yourself how many points that word is worth in Scrabble.

№ 83

Deviated Septum Surgery

SNORING CAN BE a symptom—along with nosebleeds and frequent sinus infections—of a deviated septum. That's when the cartilage that separates your nasal passages is blocked, whether due to a broken nose, since birth, or for many other reasons. A septoplasty can take care of that—but only after other methods have been exhausted.

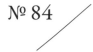

Nº 84

Rinse the Nostrils

RINSING ONE'S NOSTRILS with a saline solution—a mild decongestant—may provide some temporary snoring relief. But in the long run, it can actually be more damaging, reducing necessary defenses in the mucous membranes. So before recommending this method to your partner, consider how long of a relationship you'd actually like to have. Then act accordingly.

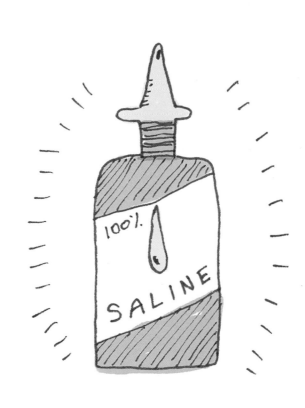

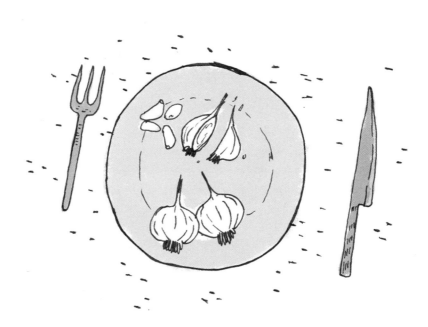

Load Up on Garlic

IF YOUR PARTNER happens to be a vampire, you might want to skip this one. If not—and if you believe in home remedies—this might be worth a shot. The theory is that garlic helps dry up nasal passages and reduce tonsil size. Whatever the case, garlic is good for you, so it won't do you any harm to factor it into dinner.

№ 86

Cannabis

AT LEAST ONE study has shown that THC—the active ingredient in marijuana—helps regulate the breathing of sleep apnea patients, although not as effectively as a CPAP or many other methods. Others advise avoiding cannabis since it can relax the throat muscles and prevent the sleeper from plunging into deeper REM sleep. This contradictory advice doesn't change the possibility that indulging in some recreational toking could help YOU get through the night.

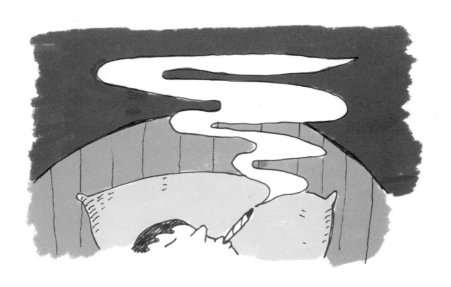

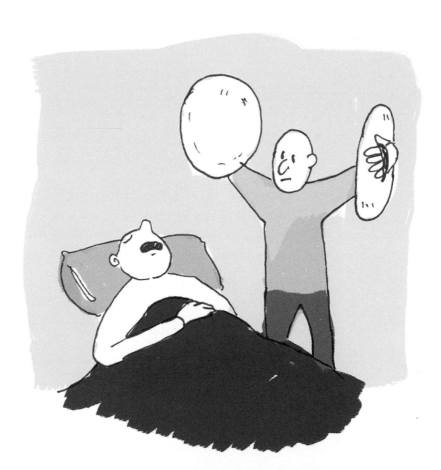

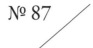

Wake the Snorer Up

YES, OF COURSE, snoring isn't the snorer's fault. And you don't want to be rude or anything. You're a good, sensitive person who only wants the best for everyone. But sometimes options are limited, sleep is necessary, and the only answer is a sensitive but firm "WAKE UP!" so that you can get some shuteye. Nobody's judging you. This might actually be your first reaction—especially if you've just been woken up by the offending noisemaker. Of course, waking them up certainly offers a temporary solution. But it also could lead to the snorer trying to engage you in conversation, turning on the TV, restlessly trying to find a new comfy spot, or otherwise distracting you from the task at hand—getting some sleep. Think before you shake.

№ 88

Massage with Mustard Oil

CREDITED WITH BEING able to help with the common cold, coughs, and more, mustard oil is also purported by some, including the folks at diyhealthremedy.com, to reduce snoring once massaged into the skin.

№ 89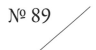

Snoring Alarm

DESIGNED TO WAKE the snorer up, these devices go off whenever they register a loud noise. The more partner-friendly ones use a vibrating patch instead of an alarm. Either way, this solution is more helpful in proving that a person actually snores than it is in addressing the problem. But awareness can be a valuable first step.

№ 90

Breath Synchronization

IMITATING THE INHALES and exhales of your snoring partner can serve as a kind of meditation that rhythmically lulls you to sleep. If it doesn't get you to nod off, it still works as a relaxation technique.

Silent Partner

USING NOISE-CANCELLATION TECHNOLOGY, this battery-operated device looks like sandbags hanging on both sides of the nose. It doesn't help the snorer, but it does attempt to cancel out the sound by emitting a counter-sound when it detects snoring. The manufacturer claims that it does its job even if you are as close as eight inches away.

№ 92

Antihistamines

IF ONE'S SNORING is accompanied by sniffling, it could be a sign that allergies are the root cause. Allergic rhinitis increases inflammation and mucus production, causing swollen airways. If that's the case, antihistamines should do the trick.

Enter the Snoratorium

A NEW WORD entered the general public's lexicon when word came out that Tom Cruise not only has a bad snoring problem but also equips his abode with a soundproof chamber for particularly loud evenings. Rumor? Perhaps. But such rooms are a reality for the rich.

№ 94

Acupressure Rings

YOU'LL BE FORGIVEN for your skepticism here. These adjustable rings—available in various sizes—go on the snorer's pinky finger 30 minutes before bedtime. Protrusions on the inside of the ring stimulate the nerve cells that are usually dormant during sleep. Bonus: If it doesn't work, you at least have some jewelry.

№ 95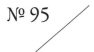

Anti-Snoring Throat Sprays

THERE IS A wide variety of throat sprays on the market with such names as SnoreStop and Snorix, all claiming to ease snoring by lubricating the throat tissues that fight mucous buildup. Consumer reviews are all over the place, from "worthless" to "life-changing." See for yourself!

№ 96

Avoid Taking Naps

WHILE IT'S TEMPTING for a snorer's partner to grab a siesta during the day to make up for lost time, those short sleep sessions could exacerbate the problem. Nodding off during the day won't have any impact on the snorer, but if you go the distance from wake-up until bedtime you may find it easier to fall asleep at night.

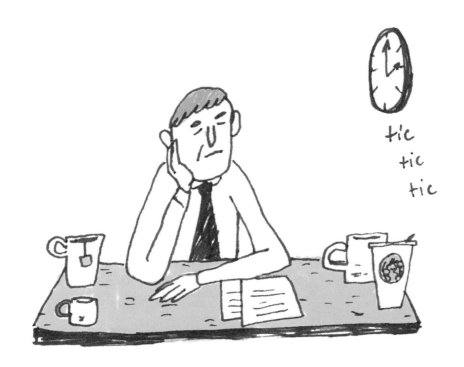

tic
tic
tic

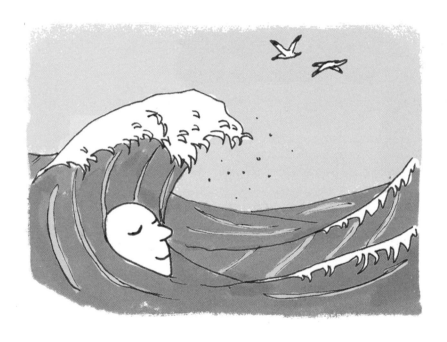

№ 97

Embrace the Snore . . . Through Hypnosis

ON A 2014 segment of the Today Show, doctors suggested some attitude adjustment on the part of the snore victim—with a little help. "Most people like sleeping next to the sound of waves," said the doc. "The snoring also comes in waves. So through hypnosis, you can give people the suggestion that every time they hear their spouse snore, it lulls them into deeper sleep."

№ 98

Record the Snorer

THE SAME TODAY Show segment that suggested hypnosis also suggested recording the snorer. This isn't intended to deal directly with the snoring but instead to prove to the snorer how loud and disturbing their nocturnal sounds are. Hopefully it will prove to them that they need to do something about it.

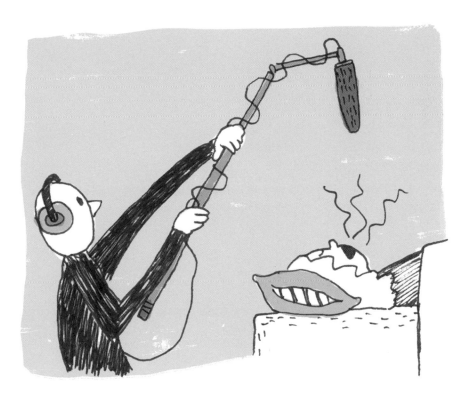

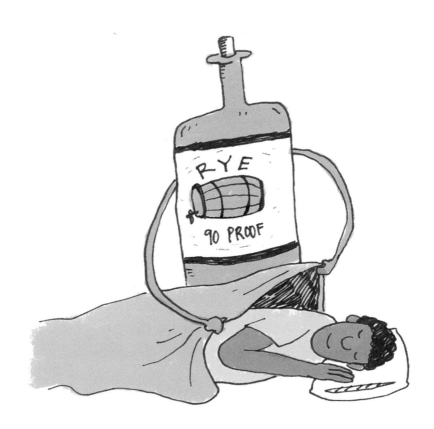

№ 99

Have a Drink . . . Or Two

DRINKING ONESELF INTO oblivion isn't a solution for the snorer and it shouldn't be one for you, either. But on a particularly difficult night when the snoring becomes unbearable, a drink may help you relax enough to nod off.

№ 100

Say a Prayer

THERE'S NO SCIENCE involved in this one, but if you buy into the idea—as many do—that divine intervention is possible and that the deity you pay homage to has enough free time and interest to deal with you and your partner's sleep issues, then by all means give this a shot. If nothing else, it could help you find the inner peace necessary to deal with that which may be out of your control. Side note: If you happen to be Catholic, look into having a chat with St. Elijah, the patron saint of sleep.

№ 101

Remind Yourself of the Truth of the Situation

AND THAT TRUTH is that snoring is not a personal failing or a deliberate effort to keep you from getting the shuteye you deserve. It's a medical condition. However many of the previous 100 methods you go through in order to find what works, remember that your bed partner isn't to blame. Good luck.

Good night!

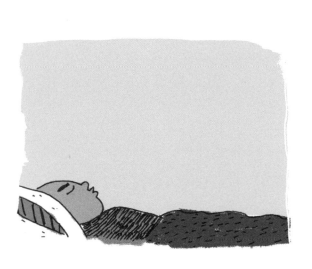

AMERICAN ACADEMY OF SLEEP MEDICINE

www.aasmnet.org

The American Academy of Sleep Medicine (AASM) works with medical professionals in order to improve sleep and individualized care amongst its practicing professionals. Offering a wide range of resources, specialized funding, and industry guidelines for professionals, the AASM's missions is to improve patient care.

AMERICAN SLEEP APNEA ASSOCIATION

www.sleepapnea.org

Founded in 1990, the American Sleep Apnea Association promotes sleep apnea awareness and healthy sleep habits through patient-led support groups and educational seminars.

AMERICAN SLEEP ASSOCIATION

www.sleepassociation.org

The American Sleep Association works closely with medical professions, patients, and other sleep organizations in order to raise awareness surrounding sleep disorders and the importance of a good night's sleep.

A.W.A.K.E.

Hosted by the American Sleep Apnea Association, the A.W.A.K.E. Network is a group comprised of those who have successfully found ways to reduce snoring. Offering publications and support to participants, A.W.A.K.E. chapters are active all across the country and are always looking for new members and chapters.

BRITISH SNORING & SLEEP APNOEA ASSOCIATION

www.britishsnoring.co.uk

Formed in 1991, the British Snoring & Sleep Apnoea Association (BSSAA) formed in order to help both snorers and sleep partners get a better night's rest. Offering helpful resources and treatments, the BSSAA works hand-in-hand with medical professionals in order to provide the most helpful information to its clients.

MAYO CLINIC

www.mayoclinic.org Based in Arizona, Florida, and Minnesota, the Mayo Clinic offers helpful resources, treatments, and care to those experiencing sleep apnea. Featuring the most up-to-date medical information surrounding sleep apnea, the Mayo Clinic is a must-see for anyone considering treatment.

SLEEPHEALTH

Working with IBM, the American Sleep Apnea Association's mobile application helps users identify and incorporate sleeping habits that will improve physical and emotional help.

SLEEP EDUCATION

www.sleepeducation.org With more than 2,500 American Academy of Sleep Medicine-accredited sleep centers in the United States, Sleep Education makes it easier than ever to connect patients with centers. Here you'll find up-to-date information on sleep disorders, as well as helpful information

surrounding treatment and incorporating better sleep habits into your life.

THE SNORING CENTER

www.snoringcenter.com The Snoring Center is a Dallas-based health clinic that offers evaluations and treatments to patients suffering from chronic snoring and sleep apnea. Founded by Dr. Craig Schwimmer, The Snoring Center understands the severity of sleep apnea and works with patients to provide individualized support.

Sleep Diary

	Sunday	Monday	Tuesday
Bedtime			
# of Times Woken			
Total Time Asleep			
Snorer Symptoms			
Techniques Used			

Wednesday	Thursday	Friday	Saturday

Sleep Diary

	Sunday	Monday	Tuesday
Bedtime			
# of Times Woken			
Total Time Asleep			
Snorer Symptoms			
Techniques Used			

Wednesday	Thursday	Friday	Saturday

Sleep Diary

	Sunday	Monday	Tuesday
Bedtime			
# of Times Woken			
Total Time Asleep			
Snorer Symptoms			
Techniques Used			

Wednesday	Thursday	Friday	Saturday

About the
Author

Lou Harry is the author of more than 30 books including *The High-Impact Infidelity Diet: A Novel*, *Creative Block*, *Kid Culture*, and *Office Dares*. His writing has appeared in publications ranging from *Men's Health* to *The Sondheim Review*. By day, he serves as Arts & Entertainment Editor for the *Indianapolis Business Journal* (www.ibj.com/arts). By night, he uses a CPAP machine.

Find him online at www.louharry.com.

About the
Illustrator

Alex Kalomeris is an illustrator, animator, printmaker, and all around storyteller. His work revolves around creating narratives, characters, and impressions. Nautical, natural, and nostalgic themes show up in his work and are an integral part of his identity as an artist. If he cannot be found in his studio, he is probably out wandering the forests and hills of his home.

Find him online at www.alexkalomeris.com.

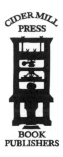

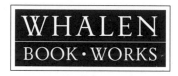

NEW YORK CITY, NEW YORK

"Where Good Books Are Ready for Press"
Good ideas ripen with time. From seed to harvest, Cider Mill Press brings fine reading, information, and entertainment together between the covers of its creatively crafted books. Our Cider Mill bears fruit twice a year, publishing a new crop of titles each spring and fall.

Whalen Book Works is a book packaging company that combines top-notch design, unique formats, and fresh content to create truly innovative gift books. We plant one tree for every 10 books we print, and your purchase supports a tree in the Rocky Mountain National Park.

Visit us on the web at
www.cidermillpress.com
or write to us at
PO Box 454, 12 Spring St.
Kennebunkport, Maine 04046

Visit us on the web at
www.whalenbooks.com
or write to us at
338 E 100 Street, Suite 5A
New York, NY 10029